Gluten Free Fitness

Beginners Guide to 10 Tasty Diet Meals to Lose Weight

By Scott Jay Marshall II

I0429368

What You Are Going To Learn

In this book I am going to tell you about 10 of THE BEST meals for anyone on a gluten free diet that I personally used to LOSE 60 LBS.! This is for those people out there trying to lose weight, keep calories low, or simply enjoy a healthy lifestyle. I'm not a ghost writer and I'm not a random guy picking a profitable subject to write about. I am a gluten intolerant man myself and have been living this lifestyle for years. I've done it the unhealthy way and the healthy way. Since you purchased this book, I know you've made the right decision and have decided to make healthy changes in your life. You'll learn about the foods you need to make these meals, as well as, a little bit of background on each item. Also, you'll discover how to prepare these items and how much of these items to have. Furthermore, you'll read how to serve these dishes and even visit a key factor to weight loss and a healthy lifestyle overall, calories. In general, the media, world, and people make losing weight and living a healthy lifestyle way more complicated than it should be. Especially when factoring in special dietary needs like gluten free (GF) eating. These meals are super easy to prepare with simple, 100% gluten free ingredients packed full of goodness.

Disclaimer

This book was written as a suggestive guide to creating healthy meals and losing weight with 100% gluten free foods. Before starting this or any other diet/weight loss program speak with your physician. The writer, distributors, and all others involved with this book are not responsible for any negative results that manifest from following the suggestions in this work. Please ensure you are buying high quality, healthy, and clean produce and foods to ensure you do not contract a foodborne illness. Always sanitize your food prep area before preparing these meals. Starting with high-quality ingredients in a sanitary environment is crucial, especially when preparing meats and other perishable food items. Lastly, inspect the cooking surfaces and tools you will use before use to ensure they are sanitary and functioning properly.

Table Of Contents

What You Are Going To Learn
Disclaimer
Table Of Contents
A Special Thank You - Free Gift
Why Should You Trust What I'm Telling You?
What Is Gluten And What Is A Gluten Free Diet?
Quick Tip/Tool/Trick
Complete Ingredient List
 Meats & Eggs:
 Fruits & Veggies:
 Other:
A Quick Word On Amounts
Meal # 1 - Steak & Taters
Meal # 2 - Fish & Veggies
Meal # 3 - The Gobbler Burger Special
Meal # 4 - Piggy & Beans
Meal # 5 - Author's Choice
Meal # 6 - The Fitness Classic
Meal # 7 - Patties, Greens & Skinny Sweets
Meal # 8 - Buff N' Stuff Breakfast
Meal # 9 - Greens, Eggs & No Ham
Meal # 10 - I Woke Up Late
A Quick Word On Meal Prepping
Conclusion
A Favor To Ask
Again, A Special Thank You
I Dedicate This Book...
About The Author

A Special Thank You - Free Gift

As a special thank you for purchasing my book, I would like to give you my irreplaceable guide to 5 of the most commonly overlooked foods containing gluten. These 5 foods get gluten free folks in trouble thousands of times a day, every day, all over the world. This is mostly because you would never think about them containing gluten.

So please accept my free gift, *The Hidden Gluten Report*. Make sure YOU know 5 of the most commonly overlooked glutinous foods on the market. You'll thank yourself for it and you'll be able avoid these major downfalls in your gluten free diet. Without this report you may eat them tomorrow, the next day, or maybe even today. This amazing report is FREE so don't miss out and take the risk of eating these glutinous foods. Unfortunately, it won't be free forever, so claim your copy now.

Claim Your FREE Copy

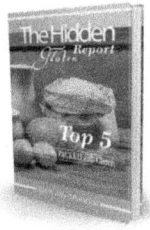

Just to give you a heads up, you'll be asked for your email address. I ask for 2 reasons:
1) So I know where to send your FREE gift.

2) 2) You're obviously an intelligent, diet minded individual living a gluten free lifestyle or trying to help someone close to you. With this in mind, I will periodically send out email notifications about additional free promotions, valuable gluten free information and discounts on my other gluten free books in the *Gluten Free Fitness* series. I NEVER spam and will always respect, and keep your email private.

Download Your FREE Copy Of "The Hidden Gluten Report"

Why Should You Trust What I'm Telling You?

Hey, that's a fair question, right? "Who's this guy telling me what's what about gluten?" On May 3, 2008, at approximately 11:30PM was the first time my gluten allergy surfaced. Some people say stressful situations make the allergy finally manifest, some say physical trauma. Whatever it was, that's when mine started. I didn't know what was going on at first so I continued to compound the problem over the coming months. At the time, I had a high amount of gluten in my diet—burgers, cereals, glutinous alcohol, chips, chicken strips, toast, you name it. Foods with gluten in them were my favorite kinds of food and I ate them all the time. With all of these compounding problems working against me problems came on quick and didn't go away until I changed my diet. I was constipated, had low energy levels, lost weight because my body wasn't getting the nutrition it needed and more.

My quality of life and health were not good.

Then, a friend with Celiac disease casually mentioned symptoms he experienced after eating gluten. They were too familiar to ignore at that point. We looked up a list of issues related to gluten allergies and found I had 18 out of 20 symptoms. So, I started eating gluten free or at least close to it. I was so new to this diet that I didn't know what had gluten in it except for the obvious items like bread. As any Celiac or gluten free dieter eventually learns, it's hidden in foods you would never expect to have it. I'll tell you more about that later.

Slowly, my health improved. The more disciplined I became with my diet the better I felt. I started gaining healthy weight back, constipation was no longer a problem, and I didn't feel super tired anymore.

Life started getting better and my health grew alongside it.

I didn't return fully to normal until I had completely cut gluten out of my diet, and even then it took awhile to get it out of my system.

Years later, I gained weight and finally decided to start eating better for good. Just because you eat gluten free doesn't mean you are consuming healthy food. So I researched and learned how to eat gluten free while staying healthy. Many of the health foods on the market or ingredients in supposedly healthy recipes have gluten (i.e. noodles, grains, granola bars, etc.). At first, it seemed like someone was asking me to dig the car out of the snow with a spoon—painful and tedious. However, after a lot of studying, I found it was actually quite easy to eat healthy and gluten free simultaneously.

You can't have the donuts or sugary cereals the company brings in for breakfast. And, you should avoid the five pieces of cake and cookie dough ice cream at any birthday party.

Before long, I had lost 60 pounds, was much happier, had started putting on muscle, and was looking lean.

At long last, my health and quality of life had reached what I would describe as nothing short of amazing.

I want to share what I learned with other people wanting to follow a gluten free diet. You can have AMAZING meals, keep calories low, not sacrifice taste or enjoyment, support a healthy weight loss plan, and do it 100% gluten free.

In short, that's why you should trust what I'm telling you. I've walked the walk and talked the talk when it comes to eating and being physically fit on a gluten free diet. Like any other healthy lifestyle, it takes commitment, discipline, and drive. You will find a gluten free lifestyle is far beyond worth it.

I'm going to assume since you bought this book, you have goals aligned with living a healthy lifestyle, enjoying satisfying food, losing some weight, and doing it gluten free. I'm here to tell you, I believe in you and know you can do it.   series and beyond.

What Is Gluten And What Is A Gluten Free Diet?

Gluten is a mixture of different proteins found in wheat and other related grains. Some refer to gluten as a "binding protein" because it often gives bread and other products it's chewy texture and feel. For example, take a raw piece of wheat, get it wet, and grind it between your fingers. You would find it produces a white, sticky substance—also known as gluten.

 A gluten free diet consists of a meal plan comprised of items 100% void of the protein(s) known as gluten. This is sometimes difficult for many reasons:

1. Wheat is cheap and is used as a filler for many different products. It is also added as a thickening agent in some foods.

2. As a direct result of #1, gluten free items can be expensive if the food item you are buying is traditionally made with gluten. Bread and soups would be a good example of those types of items. A standard loaf of gluten free bread can cost as much as $6 or more.

3. Some food companies are tricky when it comes to labeling what is in their food. For example, if you look at a bottle of Powerade you are not going to see wheat anywhere on the label. However, if you read the ingredients list of some of the flavors you will find an item called modified food starch. This is a nonspecific starch comprised of nonspecific items. Many Celiacs

report discomfort and negative reactions after they consume modified food starch because one of the most common nonspecific food items used to make it is wheat.

4. You'd be surprised to know what foods actually contain gluten. For example, many brands of jerky contain gluten. It helps the flavor stick to and impregnate the meat better which helps with flavor while it sits on the shelf.

5. For all these reasons a celiac or someone following a gluten free diet has to become a label reader which some people find exhausting. In all honesty, it can be difficult but if you are following a gluten free diet it is something you will have to get used to.

It's easy to understand why so many people feel so lost when they discover they are a Celiac or are gluten intolerant and HAVE to go on a gluten free diet. However, once you learn the basics, and get a little experience under your belt it becomes second nature.

Quick Tip/Tool/Trick

If you're serious about losing weight, monitoring calories you eat is critical. Nothing does that better than a phone app like "LoseIt!" or "MyFitnessPal." I'm not paid by anyone to mention these apps so know that I'm only telling you this information because I believe they are valuable tools. I personally use "LoseIt!" but I have heard nothing but good things about "MyFitnessPal." Both applications essentially function the same way.

They are fast, simple, straight forward, have MASSIVE databases of foods, and will really help you keep on track and stay accountable. Even better, you can scan the barcodes of the foods you eat and they will automatically calculate the calories for you instead of having to manually search and enter foods you eat. They will even give you counts on nutrients like protein, carbs, fats, and more. The best part— THEY ARE TOTALLY FREE.

The late, great Greg Plitt (an extremely influential fitness model and motivational speaker) once said if you expend more calories than you take in, YOU WILL lose weight. CLICK HERE TO WATCH THE VIDEO. What did he mean? Let's say you are eating 2500 calories a day to maintain your current weight. If you decrease it to 2300 calories a day while maintaining the same activity levels, the pounds will come off. It's an inarguable fact that works to your benefit because it's easy to track and it's guaranteed.

So do yourself a favor, go download a calorie tracking app and make the most out of your day and these meals. Seriously go, I'll be here when you get back.

LET'S GET COOKING!

Complete Ingredient List

This is a complete list of all the ingredients you will be using to put together these meals, as well as, a small tidbit about what makes each of these foods great.

Meats & Eggs:

- Trimmed Beef Sirloin
  - Beef is a classic protein source. It gets a bad rap because it is a red meat. Truthfully, it can be extremely good for you. Especially if you trim and cook a lean cut like sirloin with healthy oils (i.e. coconut oil). What do I mean by trimming? I imply to trim off the fat. For example, in the center of a sirloin steak is a "divider," where the steak breaks in half. Trim the connecting those two pieces and any fat on the outsides of the cut as well. If you have dogs, toss the trimmings to them, they'll thank you for it.
- Trimmed Pork Sirloin
  - Like beef, pork often gets a bad rap and in many cases for good reason. It IS higher in fat than other protein sources. However, you can take steps much like those steps I mentioned with beef to ensure you are getting the leanest protein possible while still allowing variety into your healthy lifestyle. Just like the beef, choosing a cut like a sirloin is ideal. It's already the more lean cut but you can also decrease the fat by trimming and cooking in healthy oils.
- Ground Turkey Burger

- While I have seen turkey burger come in ratios as fatty as 73/27 (73% meat, 27% fat), turkey burger is exceptionally lean and tasty. It's one of my favorites and I have seen it as lean as 93/7. You'll want to watch it closely while cooking if you use that ratio as the lower fat ratios burn easily because of less moisture. That's where a good healthy oil comes in. If I feel like biting into a cheesy taco but don't want to overindulge and go over my calories for the day, I make a nice batch of turkey burger tacos. They are a staple around my house.
- Lean Ground Beef Burger
    - Choosing to use a lean ratio and drain the fat from the pan as you are cooking your beef burger can make it a superior high source of protein. And, let's face it, a burger is just plain delicious.
- Chicken Breasts
    - Big surprise right? Anyone who has seen a picture of a fitness meal prep or heard someone talking about eating healthy, the chicken breast was involved for good reason. Virtually no carbs or fats, and more than 5 grams of protein per ounce. BAM! If that's not a fitness yummy, I don't know what is.
- Chicken Thighs
    - Some people suggest darker chicken meats like thighs and drumsticks can be ideal for athletes. The reason? Breast tends to be much more expensive than thighs and drumsticks because it's the staple/ideal white chicken meat everyone loves. Besides cost, the fat is another reason. Right about now you're saying, "Wait back up,

fats? I thought fats were bad." No, they are not. They are a necessity. While fats are broken down too slowly to be used as energy during workouts, they are an essential piece of all hormone production. In short, if you are a gal, fat helps you produce and maintain healthy estrogen levels. If you're a bro, the same goes for you but with testosterone as opposed to estrogen. Check out THIS ARTICLE from www.livestrong.com to learn more.

- Fish
  - It's hard to make a bad choice when it comes to fish. While salmon is, of course, the fitness food of choice, fish in general are high in protein, have virtually no carbs, and are low in bad fats. THIS ARTICLE from *Men's Journal* suggests that the best fish are salmon, albacore tuna, mackerel, and trout. So, bust out the fishing pole fisherman and catch yourself a fitness dinner!

- Turkey Sausage Patties (pre-cooked)
  - Turkey sausage is not only lower in fat, and calories than pork sausage but it tastes amazing. At this point in my life, I prefer it. With the right spices, it tastes the same as pork sausage and isn't anywhere near as greasy. I hate the feeling of tasting more grease than meat at breakfast.

- Eggs
  - Eggs, as some would say, are nature's perfect food. There is a lot of debate about cholesterol, so if that concerns you, just have egg whites instead. Separating the yolk from the white is easy enough when you crack it or you can simply buy egg whites.

Fruits & Veggies:

- Russet Potatoes
  - A staple of any table, russet potatoes are cheap, hearty, and filling.
- Red Potatoes
  - Red potatoes are the bees knees of potatoes. They are naturally gluten free, fat-free, help with energy levels, blood pressure, and even stress. Not to mention they taste excellent.
- Sweet Potatoes
  - Some call sweet potatoes one of the world's healthiest foods. It's packed full of vitamins and minerals, has an almost sweet taste, and is inexpensive.
- Granny Smith Apple
  - Truly the apple of the fitness world. Protein and fiber in one shot, they contain vitamins, minerals, antioxidants and even fight some digestive disorders. Plus, they're tasty.
- Kale
  - I LOVE kale. Yup, kale, the plant some people think is only for decoration. Often associated with a bitter taste, kale is often referred to as a superfood. It's hard to eat it the wrong way if you are into the green tasting foods. I prefer my kale raw, or blended in a smoothie with fruit and protein.
- Spinach
  - Another super food of the greens world. There is a reason they had the classic cartoon character Popeye munching this stuff down. Spinach is packed full of all the powerful things you would

expect from a green superfood but is much milder in taste compared to kale.

- Bell Peppers
  - Bell peppers come in a multitude of colors and sizes but are all basically the same. They are not hot at all as some people would suspect with "pepper" in the name. They have a very mild flavor in fact.
- Green Beans
  - Green beans belong in any fitness meal plan. Also known as string beans, they are extremely beneficial for you and even promote bone health. Not something you'd expect from a vegetable, I know.
- Broccoli
  - Broccoli is actually a member of the cabbage family. High in fiber and protein, broccoli was one of Thomas Jefferson's favorites.
- Cauliflower
  - Cauliflower is an amazing plant both for its health benefits and alternative uses. I suggest you look up "garlic cheese bread from cauliflower." You can thank me after your taste buds chill out.
- Carrots
  - One of my personal favorites, carrots are packed with beta-carotene which our bodies turn into Vitamin A. In fact, it's one of the best sources for Vitamin A in the world which is why they are so good for our vision, bones, and teeth.
- Asparagus
  - Another personal favorite, yes, really. That weird vegetable that makes your pee smell funny. Three years after planting, asparagus reaches

it's growing season and can grow as much as 6 inches PER DAY.

- Strawberries
  - Strawberries taste fantastic and are one of the best sources of antioxidants in the world.
- Blueberries
  - Full of fiber and perfect in a muffin, blueberries are excellent for you and are exceptionally tasty. They are also a strong source of antioxidants. This fruit CAN be expensive if you buy them at the wrong time of year.
- Bag of Greens
  - A mixed bag of greens will be used. This can be whatever tickles your fancy—Asian mix or power greens to name a couple.
- Banana
  - Not just for monkeys, bananas are one of the best sources of potassium around. Keep them on hand if you commonly experience charley horses in your muscles and you'll find that come less often. They are also ideal for an energy boost and sustained blood sugar levels right before a workout.
- Cucumber
  - Cucumbers taste crisp and clean, are extremely inexpensive, and are basically tubes of water with skin so they are an awesome choice to add to salads or eat in slices to help with hydration.

Other:

- Protein Powder

- A must-have for anyone going through strenuous workouts. For approximately 45 minutes after a workout, your body is going to be screaming for protein to put the muscle fibers you just tore back together. Absorbing protein in liquid form via protein shakes allows your body to digest it faster and easier which means your body gets more out of it when it needs it most.
- Instant Oatmeal
  - Often overlooked in fitness and diets, oatmeal is full of fiber and extremely tasty when you add cinnamon or fruits. Instant oatmeal is better if you are going to use it in the morning when time is short. And, there are TONS of gluten free instant oatmeal on the market that taste excellent.
- Cinnamon
  - Cinnamon helps sustain healthy insulin levels, has anti-inflammatory properties, has been linked to heart disease prevention, is full of antioxidants, fights several types of infections, and the list goes on. Cinnamon is one those spices you should keep in your diet at all times. If you don't enjoy the flavor, it does come in capsule form.
- Yogurt
  - What type you get is totally up to you. Greek yogurt, plain, key lime, some type of fruit yogurt—it's hard to go wrong with a good yogurt. The best kinds will come with live, active cultures for your digestive system.
- White Rice
  - White rice is inexpensive, goes with almost anything, and is extremely low in calories.

- Brown Rice
  - Brown rice shares the same benefits of white rice but is an even better grain choice for you. It's high in fiber, helps keep blood sugar levels in check, and studies show it supports the reduction of high cholesterol levels.
- Butter
  - Yes, butter in a diet book. People often assume that eating healthy means not eating foods you really enjoy. This is not the case. Instead, you practice control and don't go overboard. For example, I will use small amount of butter for one meal in this book.
- Lemon Juice
  - Lemon juice is inexpensive and adds a kick to a lot of different foods. It's available in all different kinds like organic, and all natural. This citrus juice can be found at almost any grocery store, and is virtually calorie free.
- Some Standard Seasonings
  - Salt, black pepper, garlic salt, onion powder, chopped and dried onions.

Now that we have our complete list of items, let's put them to good use.

A Quick Word On Amounts

I'm going to give amounts for each item of the meals. However, feel free to modify these amounts as you see fit to line up with your dietary needs and fitness goals. Just understand as you add more, the calories of the meal will increase. And, if you take food away, the calories will decrease.

LET'S GET TO IT!!!

Meal # 1 - Steak & Taters

Ingredients:

- 8 oz. trimmed beef sirloin
- 1 russet potato
- 1 sliced bell pepper
- Standard Seasonings (to taste)

Preparations:

- Rinse off your potato and poke holes in it with a fork for a faster cook time. Then wrap it in tin foil.
- Cut up your bell pepper by slicing off the top, then slicing it into quarters and removing the seeds. Finally, cut it into thin strips no more than a half-inch wide.
- Make sure your sirloin is defrosted and ready to cook. If you get caught in a jam and forget to defrost it, then you can either stick it in the microwave, or you can put it in a container of HOT water until it's defrosted. When it is defrosted, take a good sharp knife and trim off any visible fat. Yes, this may sacrifice a small amount of flavor but ultimately makes it a healthier meal.

Making The Meal:

1. Get your potato cooking first since it takes the longest to cook. You can cook it in a standard oven, a toaster oven, or as a last resort, the microwave. The first two

options will produce a much better result. Generally, a baked potato can take an hour to cook so squeeze in a workout or something else productive while it cooks. If you're using the microwave the amount of time will vary.

2. After your potato has been cooking for about 40-45 minutes in the oven, grab a healthy oil like coconut oil and throw it into a pan. It doesn't take much. Then season and cook your steak to your liking—rare, medium rare, medium well, well done. When you have 5 minutes left of cooking the steak, throw in the strips of bell pepper. This will blend the flavors of your steak and peppers. Cook the peppers long enough to still have their crisp snap.

3. To serve, slice your steak into strips and put them on a plate with your peppers so they can be eaten together in a single bite and place your baked potato on a small plate on the side. Feel free to add salt, pepper and a small amount of butter to your potato but stay away from cheese to keep things low in calories. Then, of course, enjoy.

Meal # 2 - Fish & Veggies

Ingredients:

- 1 fillet of your favorite type of fish
- 1 head of broccoli
- ½ head of cauliflower
- 2 carrots
- ¼ stick of butter
- Standard Seasonings (to taste)

Preparations:

- Rinse off your broccoli, cauliflower and carrots, as you always should with your produce.
- Make sure your fillet is defrosted and ready to be cooked.

Making The Meal:

1. Preheat your oven to around 450°F. Season your fish with lemon juice, garlic salt, onion powder, and pepper. Check your fish periodically. Depending on your oven, cook time should be between 35-45 minutes. To test the fish and make sure it is done, just stick it with a fork and see if it comes apart easily.
2. While your fish is cooking, melt a SMALL amount of butter in a dish to brush your over your broccoli and cauliflower. Then add a small amount of salt and

pepper and begin to steam them. If you don't have a steamer, then you can either stir fry the veggies in a pan with some healthy coconut oil or you could eat it raw. Raw is my personal favorite. You don't lose any of the nutrients through the cooking process and I find having a cold crisp food to counter the cooked meat is excellent.

3. To serve, combine all of the vegetables in a large bowl and place fish fillet on a small plate and enjoy.

Meal # 3 - The Gobbler Burger Special

Ingredients:

- 10-12 ounces of ground turkey burger. You will lose a lot of the weight during the cooking process like you will with any ground meat. Cooked, you'll end up with 6-8 ounces which is an ideal amount for a single serving when you are on a fitness diet. Protein is ESSENTIAL to any fitness diet.
- 1 cup of rice
- 2 carrots
- 1 handful of asparagus
- Standard Seasonings (to taste)

Preparations:

- Make sure your turkey burger is defrosted. If you forget to defrost ahead of time, turkey burger will defrost rapidly. Simply put it in hot water for a few minutes. Only until you can easily break the turkey burger apart. It's SO much easier if you have meats separated ahead of time because it allows you to defrost and manage them easily.
- Rinse and cut the tops and bottoms off of your carrots and the bottoms off of your asparagus. I like to cut my asparagus in half horizontally but I'll leave that up to you. Next, take your carrots and cut them in half, and then cut them in half long ways. I recommend a sharp

knife and SLOW, CONTROLLED movements. It's easier to cut yourself than you would think.

Making The Meal:

1. Start the rice first. If you are using 5-minute rice, then still do it first so it can be out of the way. OF COURSE, make sure while you are shopping for this white rice, you find a white rice labeled gluten free because not all white rice is gluten free.
2. Get your turkey burger cooking in a pan. This time, do not use any cooking oil. The water that is expelled from the turkey burger will be more than enough to prevent it from burning unless you are using a very lean ratio. Then a little coconut oil would be appropriate. Fair warning, turkey burger cooks much faster than beef burger so be on the lookout for that. To make sure it's done, make sure there is no amount of pink leftover in the middle or anywhere else. Poultry should always be thoroughly cooked for safety. Season with salt, onion powder, and black pepper. This isn't in the ingredient list but if you would like you can research poultry herb mixes to use as well.
3. In this recipe, the carrots and asparagus are meant to be served raw. This is one of my all time favorite lunch meals. If you would like you could steam them or throw them into the pan with your turkey burger once it has completely cooked. If you do give it a try and stay open-minded, I think you will really enjoy the combination of cooked and raw foods.
4. To serve, mix your turkey burger and rice together in a large bowl. Then place your carrots and asparagus on a small plate and dig in!

Meal # 4 - Piggy & Beans

Ingredients:

- 8 oz. of trimmed pork sirloin
- 1 cup of brown rice
- 7 oz. of green beans (approx. half of a standard can)
- Standard Seasonings (to taste)

Preparations:

- Measure 1 cup of brown rice into a bowl or cup.
- Open your can of green beans. If you're not getting it from a can then simply eyeball half of a can's worth.You can put plastic over the can and save the other half for later, or cook it all now and save the cooked portion in the fridge to be eaten later.
- Make sure your pork is defrosted. Just like I discussed with the beef sirloin, you are going to want to trim your pork sirloin. Typically, the pork sirloin will be fattier than the beef sirloin so you are going to have more to trim. Again, practice safety, and use a sharp knife to carefully do your trimming.

Making The Meal:

1. Prepare your rice in a rice cooker first. Brown rice generally takes longer to cook than white rice so follow the directions on the package you bought. Also, make sure you buy a brand specifically marked gluten free.

Just like I discussed with white rice, not all brown rice brands on the market are gluten free. So, do your research and make sure it's gluten free before you waste your money and buy it. This shouldn't be difficult. Labeling foods as gluten free has become a strong marketing point for food manufacturers and producers.

2. Put your beans in a pot with water and start cooking them on a medium heat until they are soft and break easily with a spoon or fork.

3. While your rice and beans cook, pull out a pan and melt some healthy oil like coconut oil down in the pan. Pork has a tendency to stick to the pan so make sure you cover the entire pan surface with the oil. Pork should be cooked THOROUGHLY. Season with garlic salt, onion powder, black pepper, chopped and dried onions. If you decided to research poultry herb mixes give that a shot as well. Mmm, delicious!

4. Serve everything together on a single plate and enjoy.

Meal # 5 - Author's Choice

Ingredients:

- 2-3 medium sized chicken thighs. Chicken loses a lot of it's weight during the cooking process and you want to end up with approximately 8 oz. of cooked chicken which the 2-3 thighs should provide.
- 1 cucumber
- 1 carrot
- 1 large or 2 medium sized red potato(es)
- Standard Seasonings (to taste)
- Cinnamon

Preparations:

- Rinse off the cucumber, carrot, and potatoes.
- Cut the tip and bottom off the carrot and slice it diagonally into circular slices.
- Slice your red potatoes into 8 pieces. To do this, cut it in half and then section those 2 pieces into 4. This will make it easier to cook and will help the potato absorb any seasons you choose to add.
- Slice your cucumber horizontally into circular slices about a quarter-inch thick.
- Remove the skin from your chicken thighs. To reduce cook time, remove the bone as well and slice the chicken thigh into smaller pieces. Inch wide strips should do. If you're not that confident with a knife, you don't need to remove the bone. It will just take a little

longer to cook as the bone holds a lot of cold and takes the longest to warm up, increasing cook time.

Making The Meal:

1. Take your carrot and potatoes and put them into a pot to start cooking or put them in a steamer or crock pot. They will be done when the potatoes are soft and break easily. Depending on your cooking method this will take 30-60 minutes. Do this first since it will take the longest.
2. Your cucumber is ready so no more prep needed there.
3. Throw water into a pan and get your chicken cooking at a high heat. Like pork, you want to thoroughly cook chicken until there is no pink leftover, at all. When the meat breaks apart easily and white all the way through, then you know it is done. Make sure you continue to add water during the cooking process so the meat doesn't dry out or burn in the pan. I like to use all of the standard seasonings in this recipe. I also add a small amount of cinnamon to this recipe, cinnamon is very good for you and the salty/sweet clash is amazing.
4. To serve, place your chicken, carrot slices and potatoes on a plate with your cucumber slices in a small bowl and enjoy.

Meal # 6 - The Fitness Classic

Ingredients:

- 1 large trimmed chicken breast or 2 small trimmed chicken breasts
- 1 cup of brown rice
- 1 granny smith apple
- Standard Seasonings (to taste)

Preparations:

- Measure out 1 cup of brown rice into a bowl or cup.
- For ease of eating and presentation, cut your apple into 4 sections. Remove the stem first. Next, cut your apple into quarters. Follow up by carefully slicing from top to bottom and remove the center of each slice that contains any seeds or piece of the core. Apple seeds contain cyanide and should never, ever be eaten. It would take a large amount to make you sick but it's best to just avoid them altogether.
- Make sure that your chicken breast defrosts all the way through. With a sharp knife, remove any excess fat that is on the breast.

Making The Meal:

1. Similar to meal 4, prepare your rice in a rice cooker first. Brown rice generally takes longer to cook than white rice so follow the directions on the package you

bought. Again, make sure you use gluten free brown rice marked gluten free on the package.

2. Place a small spoonful of coconut oil or any other healthy oil that you choose into a pan and make sure it covers the entire surface of the pan. Cook the chicken breast at medium to high heat until it is white all the way through and comes apart easily. I know I'm beating a dead horse here but ALWAYS cook chicken thoroughly. Season with black pepper, onion powder, garlic salt, and a small dash of cinnamon. Trust me, it's good.

3. To serve, cut the chicken breast into strips or chunks and mix it into the brown rice with your apple slices on a small plate on the side and munch away.

Meal # 7 - Patties, Greens & Skinny Sweets

Ingredients:

- 10 oz. of lean ground beef
- Half a sweet potato
- 2 cups of spinach
- Standard Seasonings (to taste)

Preparations:

- Rinse your spinach and sweet potato.
- Cut your sweet potato in half lengthwise and either put the other half away or cook both halves now and save one for later. I recommend the latter. Potatoes do not keep well after the insides have been exposed to oxygen.
- Put your defrosted ground beef into a Ziploc bag and add your desired ratios of the standard seasonings. Now seal the bag and mash everything together. This will make clean up of your pan later much easier and will ensure even seasoning distribution. You can apply this same technique to ground turkey. Next, take your ground beef and separate it into 2 balls of equal size. Then, flatten the balls into a patty. To keep your burgers from rising into a dome when you cook them, put a small dent in the middle of each patty with your knuckle or a spoon.

Making The Meal:

1. Wrap your sweet potato in tin foil and throw it in the oven at 450°F or in your toaster oven at the same temperature. Throw it in flat side down. You will know it is done when you push on the potato and it easily sinks in. This will take 45-60 minutes depending on the size of your sweet potato and oven.

2. Place your spinach in a bowl and cover it with your favorite salad dressing or leave it as is. Feel free to add other veggies if you want but I'm restricting it to spinach to stick with the recipe.

3. Put your hamburger patties into a pan and cook to your preference—well done, medium well, and so on. There is no need to add extra seasoning since you did it earlier. After flipping your burgers for the first time, remove them and set them on a plate and drain the grease from your pan into an old coffee can or another container that won't melt. Then put your patties back into the pan and finish cooking them. This will make the meal even leaner.

4. Serve with the patties and sweet potato on a plate with your spinach in a bowl on the side and enjoy.

Meal # 8 - Buff N' Stuff Breakfast

Ingredients:

- Your favorite flavor of gluten free instant oatmeal
- Cinnamon
- 1 scoop of protein powder
- ½ cup of blueberries
- 5 strawberries
- 1 cup of kale

Preparations:

- Get your blender or magic bullet out for your shake.
- Rinse your blueberries, strawberries, and kale.
- Remove the leafy part of the kale from the stem and toss the remains.
- Using a straw (you can see videos of this on YouTube) remove the center and leaves from your strawberries. Then using a sharp knife, cut them in half. If you don't have straws on hand you can just cut and remove the center or leave the center. Just make sure you at least remove the leaves and stem from the top.

Making The Meal:

1. Following the directions on the package, cook your instant oatmeal in the microwave. When it is done, add cinnamon and stir it in thoroughly for even distribution.

2. While your oatmeal cools, put your kale, blueberries, strawberries and protein powder into your blender along with a small amount of water, it doesn't take much. If you are using a smaller bullet style blender, then blend everything except the protein powder first. Add the protein powder and do one more quick run.
3. To serve, sit down at the table with a good book or view out your window. Put your shake into a large glass, enjoy your bowl of oatmeal, and fuel your morning.

Meal # 9 - Greens, Eggs & No Ham

Ingredients:

- 2 large eggs or the equivalent amount of egg white liquid if you are going that route
- 1 cup of mixed greens
- 1 cup of water
- 1.5 cups of your favorite fruit
- 2 ice cubes (if you have sensitive teeth you can leave these out or use cold fruit)
- Salt and pepper (to taste)

Preparations:

- Rinse your greens and fruit
- Place your egg whites or eggs into a bowl. Next, add salt and pepper and mix it all together with a whisk or fork.
- Pull out your blender. (A bullet is not recommended for this meal)

Making The Meal:

1. Put your eggs or whites into a pan and cook on medium heat until done.
2. Combine and blend the water, greens, fruit, and ice if you've decided to use it into your blender.
3. Serve your eggs on a small plate with your greens/fruit shake in a tall glass and enjoy.

Meal # 10 - I Woke Up Late

Ingredients:

- 2-3 prepackaged turkey sausage patties
- 1 banana
- 1 cup of yogurt (by cup I mean a single serving like you would pack in someone's lunch)

Making The Meal:

1. This meal is designed for those mornings when you have no time to make breakfast. Following the instructions, heat the turkey sausage patties in the microwave.
2. Grab your banana and yogurt while your turkey sausage patties are heating up.
3. Wrap your turkey sausage patties in a paper towel and head out the door to start your day.

A Quick Word On Meal Prepping

These ten meals are palate pleasing and good for you but sometimes you simply don't have time to cook. Well, fret not, there is a solution. To make all of this easier, spend some time on Sundays, or any free day you have, preparing your meals for the week or, at least the meal you never have time to cook. In my case, that's lunch, which is the case for many people.

All you need to do is increase the amounts in these recipes to accommodate the number of meals you want to make. If you want to have Meal #6 for lunch during a given week, cook five chicken breasts, cut up five apples, and make five cups of rice.

Invest in a good set of Tupperware and keep Ziploc bags on hand to separate the meals. For example, If I were prepping Meal 6, then I would put a breast and cup of rice in one container and my apples in another container or Ziploc bag.

The whole point behind meal prepping is to ensure you have readily available healthy meals in line with your fitness and diet goals. This is an underutilized tool in the fitness and diet world. It's easy to justify eating out when you don't have food prepared. Especially if you live a busy lifestyle. Plus, you get to have a home cooked meal rather than crap fast food or a TV dinner for sustenance.

So, do yourself a favor, utilize these meals and make larger amounts of them ahead of time. Set yourself apart from the others out there and give yourself a fighting edge in the fitness and diet game.

Conclusion

There you have it ladies and gentlemen—*10 tasty Gluten Free Fitness meals* to help you stay on track with your diet and weight loss goals. I sincerely hope you enjoyed the first book in the *Gluten Free Fitness* series and I want to commend you. Taking control of your health, especially on a gluten free diet, is hard and takes a lot of character and drive. So congratulations! You're one of the proud folks who have decided to live a better, healthier life. You rock!

A Favor To Ask

I must ask you for a favor. If you thought this guide was valuable, please leave me a review on Amazon (CLICK HERE). It would really help me out and would help this book reach more gluten free eaters. For those readers who don't know, reviews are one of the key factors to any Kindle book's success and ranking. Also, please share it with your other gluten free friends on Facebook, Instagram, Twitter, YouTube, Periscope, Snapchat, WHEREVER!

If sharing this book could help another gluten free eater get healthy, lose weight, and become more fit, then what are you waiting for?! Sometimes the only thing people need to make big changes in their lives is a little direction and motivation from a friend. When they see the success you're having, you'll inspire them to do the same.

DON'T FORGET YOUR FREE GIFT!

Again, A Special Thank You

As I come to a close, I would like to say "Thank you!" again. All of you gluten free readers and eaters are why I wrote this book and I thank you for that.

Do yourself a favor and download "The Hidden Gluten Report" ABSOLUTELY FREE!

Click Here & Claim Your FREE Copy

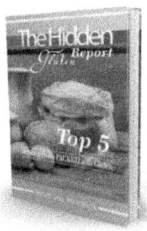

You'll learn about the 5 most commonly overlooked glutinous foods on the market. I may sound like a broken record at this point but I spent YEARS eating these without knowing I was eating gluten. It was only through extensive research, and some very uncomfortable days that I learned the truth. DON'T WAIT! It won't be free forever.

Download Your FREE Copy Of "The Hidden Gluten Report"

I Dedicate This Book…

…to the many health and fitness idols I have had over the years. My father, the late Greg Plitt, Bruce Lee, author and personal trainer Dale L. Roberts, and so many others.

As always, a dedication must go to my wonderful wife who is the foundation and core of my strength, heart, and essence. You are, and always will be, the best fan I have or will ever. I love you sweetheart.

About The Author

Scott lives amongst the purple, snow capped mountains in Northern Utah. He has lived amongst the red sand of Southern Utah as well. He lives there with his wife and 2 German Shepherds. He grew up in the area and has always had a passion for fitness. Scott is the creator of the "Doing It Better" YouTube Channel/vlog, is an avid social media buff, and loves sharing content. He loves writing about a variety of subjects including but not limited to fitness, dogs, self help, and more. He enjoys sharing stories and ideas with entrepreneurs around the world and believes that there are few people in this world that don't have something to teach, share, create, and be.

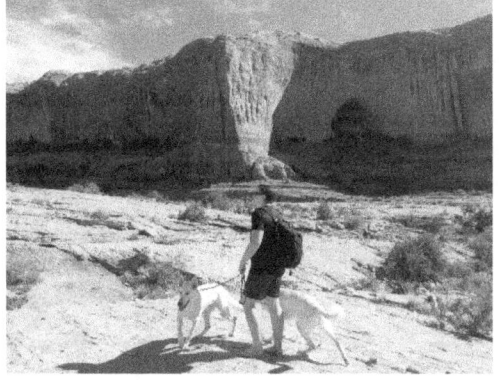

<u>Gluten Free Fitness - Beginners Guide to 10 Tasty Diet Meals to Lose Weight</u>

By Scott Jay Marshall II